TOTAL HEALING FROM GOUT: A DIET COOKBOOK FOR SENIORS AND BEGINNERS

A Simple Guide to Anti-inflammatory Relief for Weight Loss, Reducing Uric Acid Levels, and Managing Flares

Joe Miller, RD

COPYRIGHT PAGE

Table of Contents

INTRODUCTION

Gout, a form of arthritis characterized by abrupt and intense bouts of pain, swelling, and joint inflammation, has long been intertwined with dietary influences. Despite the challenges it poses, armed with knowledge and tools, individuals can assert control over their condition and enhance their overall well-being.

Total Healing from Gout: A Diet Cookbook for Seniors and Beginners is a meticulously crafted guide designed to empower individuals in navigating the complexities of gout management.

Within the pages of this comprehensive volume, we embark on an enlightening exploration of the intricate interplay between diet and gout, unraveling the nuanced role of various foods in either triggering or alleviating gout symptoms. Drawing upon cutting-edge scientific research and expert perspectives, we delve deeply into the art and science of gout management, presenting readers with actionable insights, customizable meal plans, and tantalizing recipes meticulously tailored to the unique needs of those grappling with gout.

Whether you find yourself at the outset of your gout journey, grappling with a recent diagnosis, or you've traversed its challenges for years, this book serves as your steadfast companion and roadmap to improved health and vitality. By making informed dietary decisions and embracing a holistic approach to gout care, you can reclaim agency over your life, fostering enhanced mobility, vitality, and freedom from the shackles of pain and discomfort.

Embark with us on this transformative odyssey as we set forth on a quest to conquer gout through the transformative power of nutrition and lifestyle adjustments. Together, let's take that pivotal first step toward a brighter, healthier future, emboldened by the knowledge and strategies laid forth in this indispensable guide.

CHAPTER 1
AN OVERVIEW OF THE GOUT

Gout, a form of arthritis triggered by the accumulation of uric acid crystals in the joints, presents as intense pain, swelling, and redness, often targeting the big toe. While pharmaceutical interventions and lifestyle adjustments offer avenues for gout management, the pivotal role of dietary choices cannot be overstated in both preventing and mitigating the severity of gout attacks.

At the heart of a gout diet lies the objective of lowering uric acid levels in the bloodstream. Purines, naturally occurring compounds found in certain foods, serve as the precursors to uric acid production within the body. The excruciating symptoms of gout arise from the formation of sharp urate crystals within the joints, a consequence of elevated uric acid levels.

Central to a well-crafted gout diet plan is the reduction of purine-rich foods. These often include organ meats, shellfish, red meat, and specific varieties of fish. By curtailing the intake of these purine-laden sources, the body's uric acid production diminishes, thereby reducing the likelihood of gout flare-ups and minimizing the risk of further joint deterioration.

Moreover, a gout-friendly dietary approach emphasizes the consumption of low-purine foods and beverages. Fresh fruits, vegetables, whole grains, nuts, and low-fat dairy products stand as exemplary choices for individuals grappling with gout. Beyond their low purine content, these food items are rich in essential nutrients, vitamins, minerals, and antioxidants, fostering overall health while potentially mitigating inflammation.

Hydration emerges as another cornerstone of gout management through diet. Adequate water intake facilitates the kidneys' ability to eliminate surplus uric acid from the body, thwarting its accumulation within the joints. Therefore, individuals afflicted with gout are encouraged to maintain optimal hydration levels by consuming ample water daily.

However, the intricate interplay between diet and gout necessitates a nuanced approach. Not all purine-rich foods demand complete exclusion; rather, moderation and portion control are key considerations when incorporating such items into a gout diet. A comprehensive gout management strategy extends beyond dietary adjustments, encompassing facets like weight management, regular exercise, and prudent alcohol consumption, all of which exert profound influences on gout flare-ups.

This comprehensive guide to the gout diet furnishes readers with an exhaustive exploration of the role of dietary interventions in gout management. From elucidating gout-friendly food choices to providing practical insights for crafting personalized meal plans, this resource equips individuals with the knowledge and tools essential for navigating their gout treatment journey. However, it is imperative to consult with healthcare professionals before embarking on significant dietary or treatment modifications. As you embark on this journey towards a gout-free existence characterized by enhanced well-being, remember that informed decisions, underpinned by medical guidance, pave the way for a healthier, more comfortable life.

Factors contributing to the onset of Gout

Gout, characterized by the accumulation of uric acid crystals in the joints, manifests as inflammation, discomfort, and swelling. This condition arises from the body's impaired ability to efficiently process uric acid, a natural byproduct formed during the breakdown of purines. While purines are ubiquitous in many foods, certain individuals may possess genetic predispositions or underlying health conditions hindering the elimination of uric acid, leading to its excessive presence in the bloodstream.

Central to managing gout is the adoption of a gout-friendly diet, given that certain foods rich in purines can exacerbate symptoms by elevating uric acid production. High-purine foods such as organ meats (e.g., liver, kidneys), red meats (e.g., beef, lamb, pork), shellfish, and select fish varieties (e.g., anchovies, sardines, herring) are particularly noteworthy culprits. Furthermore, beverages like beer and high-fructose sweetened drinks have been associated with increased gout risk due to their impact on uric acid levels.

In contrast, a gout-specific dietary approach emphasizes the consumption of low-purine foods to mitigate uric acid levels and reduce the frequency of gout attacks. Embracing a diet rich in fruits, vegetables, whole grains, nuts, and low-fat dairy products provides essential nutrients while minimally impacting uric acid production.

Hydration management is equally imperative in a gout diet regimen. Adequate water intake serves to dilute uric acid, thereby diminishing the likelihood of crystal formation in the joints and promoting its excretion through urine. Additionally, maintaining optimal fluid levels can help deter the formation of kidney stones, a potential consequence of uric acid accumulation in the kidneys.

Portion control and mindful food selection constitute essential components of a gout-friendly diet. Striving for dietary balance and moderation, particularly in the consumption of high-purine foods, significantly reduces the incidence of gout attacks. Furthermore, achieving and maintaining a healthy weight is pivotal, as obesity correlates with an augmented risk of gout and exacerbation of symptoms.

Given the underlying metabolic dysfunction inherent in gout, a concerted effort towards dietary modification is imperative. By prioritizing hydration and selecting foods conducive to lower uric acid levels, individuals with gout can effectively manage their condition and enhance joint health. Through informed dietary decisions and consultation with healthcare professionals or qualified dietitians, gout sufferers can proactively mitigate the impact of this condition, ultimately improving their quality of life.

Signs and manifestations of Gout

When uric acid crystals accumulate in the joints, they precipitate the onset of gout, a form of arthritis characterized by periodic bouts of intense symptoms. These gout symptoms manifest in various forms, each contributing to the discomfort and impairment experienced by individuals afflicted with this condition.

The hallmark of gout is acute joint pain, typically striking with sudden and excruciating intensity. Often localized to a single joint, most commonly the big toe, this pain can be so severe that it disrupts sleep and daily activities. Affected joints become tender to the touch, exhibiting heightened sensitivity and discomfort.

Accompanying the pain is edema and inflammation, further exacerbating the distress of gout sufferers. Swelling in the affected joint is pronounced, leading to a visible enlargement and a sensation of warmth upon touch. The inflammatory response triggered by uric acid crystals contributes to this swelling and may impede joint mobility, resulting in a reduced range of motion that adds to the challenges of daily life.

Notably, gout can also manifest in the skin surrounding the affected joint, with notable changes in appearance. Swelling may cause the skin to take on a stretched, glossy appearance, while underlying inflammation can manifest as redness or purplish discoloration. Additionally, the formation of tophi, small chalk-like lumps resulting from the accumulation of uric acid crystals under the skin, presents another characteristic feature of advanced gout.

In severe cases, gout attacks may be accompanied by systemic symptoms such as fever and chills, reflecting the body's inflammatory response to the presence of uric acid crystals. Left untreated or inadequately managed, recurrent gout attacks can lead to worsening joint damage and an increased risk of complications.

It is important to note that gout is not limited to the big toe; it can affect various joints throughout the body, including the ankles, knees, wrists, and fingers. This diversity of affected joints underscores the need for a comprehensive understanding of gout symptoms and their differential diagnosis from other forms of arthritis and joint disorders. Accurate diagnosis is crucial for initiating appropriate treatment strategies and minimizing the long-term impact of gout on joint health and overall quality of life.

CHAPTER 2
AN OVERVIEW OF THE GOUT DIET

Understanding the intricate interplay between dietary choices and the synthesis and elimination of uric acid within the body underscores the paramount importance of diet in the management of gout. Certain foods have been identified to either exacerbate or ameliorate gout symptoms by influencing uric acid levels.

Foods rich in purines, such as organ meats, red meat, shellfish, and select varieties of fish, have been associated with elevated uric acid levels in the bloodstream, thereby increasing the risk of gout attacks. These purine-rich foods contribute to the production of uric acid, overwhelming the body's capacity to eliminate it efficiently, consequently leading to the crystallization of urate crystals in the joints, precipitating painful gout flares.

Conversely, the consumption of low-purine foods presents a promising avenue for mitigating gout symptoms and reducing the frequency of gout attacks. Fresh fruits and vegetables, whole grains, and low-fat dairy products are among the dietary staples that have been shown to aid in lowering uric acid levels in the body. These nutrient-rich foods not only provide essential vitamins, minerals, and antioxidants but also support optimal metabolic function, promoting the efficient excretion of uric acid from the body.

By strategically incorporating low-purine foods into one's diet while minimizing the intake of purine-rich fare, individuals with gout can proactively manage their condition and mitigate the associated symptoms. Moreover, adopting a well-balanced diet that aligns with the principles of gout management offers a holistic approach to health and well-being, addressing not only the immediate symptoms of gout but also contributing to overall health optimization and disease prevention.

In essence, the role of diet in gout management extends far beyond mere sustenance; it serves as a potent tool in modulating uric acid levels and attenuating the impact of gout on one's quality of life. By making informed dietary choices and embracing a gout-friendly diet rich in low-purine foods, individuals can empower themselves to take control of their health and effectively manage the challenges posed by this chronic condition.

Foods and Drinks Suitable for Individuals with Gout

Low-Purine Foods: Gout, characterized by the accumulation of uric acid in the bloodstream, resulting in the formation of crystals within joints and subsequent pain and inflammation, can be significantly influenced by dietary choices. Central to gout management is the regulation of purine intake, as purines metabolize into uric acid within the body. Opting for low-purine foods is a cornerstone strategy in mitigating uric acid levels and minimizing gout flare-ups.

Fortunately, a plethora of nutrient-rich options exists within the realm of low-purine foods. Fruits, vegetables, whole grains, and plant-based protein sources such as tofu and legumes emerge as dietary allies in this endeavor. These foods not only provide essential nutrients but also tend to have lower purine content, thus offering a balanced approach to nutrition without exacerbating gout symptoms.

Conversely, high-purine foods pose a considerable risk for gout sufferers. Items such as organ meats, certain shellfish, red meats, and select poultry varieties are notorious for their purine-rich profiles. While complete elimination of these foods may not be necessary, moderation is key. By reducing both the frequency and portion sizes of high-purine fare, individuals can better manage their uric acid levels and mitigate the likelihood of gout attacks.

Protein, an essential component of any diet, warrants special consideration in the context of gout management. While animal proteins high in purines should be consumed sparingly, alternatives abound. Lean poultry, plant-based proteins, and omega-3-rich fish offer gout-friendly substitutions that not only contribute to dietary diversity but also support overall health and well-being.

Fruits and vegetables form the bedrock of a gout-friendly diet, owing to their low-purine content and myriad health benefits. Beyond their anti-inflammatory properties, certain fruits like cherries have garnered attention for their potential to alleviate gout symptoms. Colorful, nutrient-dense options such as berries, oranges, spinach, and bell peppers further bolster gout control by virtue of their antioxidant-rich profiles.

Whole grains emerge as stalwart allies in the quest for gout management, providing a rich source of low-purine carbohydrates. Unlike their refined counterparts, whole grains boast higher fiber content and a lower glycemic index, factors that contribute to improved digestion and blood sugar regulation. By incorporating whole grains like brown rice, oats, and quinoa into their diets, individuals can enhance both their overall health and their ability to manage gout-related symptoms.

Dairy products, particularly low-fat varieties, offer unique benefits in gout management. Rich in calcium and protein, dairy products like milk, yogurt, and cheese contribute to bone health and may help lower uric acid levels. Furthermore, compounds such as casein and orotic acid found in dairy products have been associated with uric acid reduction, further underscoring their value in a gout-friendly diet.

Hydration plays a pivotal role in gout management, as adequate fluid intake facilitates the elimination of excess uric acid from the body. Water reigns supreme as the optimal hydrating agent, while herbal teas featuring anti-inflammatory ingredients like ginger and turmeric offer additional benefits. While coffee consumption has been linked to decreased uric acid levels, alcohol intake, particularly of beer and spirits, should be moderated due to its potential to exacerbate gout symptoms.

In essence, the pursuit of effective gout management necessitates a multifaceted approach, with dietary choices serving as a linchpin in the endeavor. By prioritizing low-purine foods, emphasizing nutrient-rich options, and incorporating gout-friendly substitutions, individuals can take proactive steps towards managing their condition and improving their overall quality of life.

The Significance of Incorporating Fruits and Vegetables into One's Diet

In the realm of gout management, the pivotal role of fruits and vegetables cannot be overstated, as these nutritional powerhouses offer a multitude of health benefits that extend far beyond their mere culinary appeal. Their inherent richness in essential nutrients, coupled with their relatively low purine content, renders them indispensable allies in the ongoing battle against gout and the associated risks of uric acid accumulation and flare-ups.

Fruits and vegetables, renowned for their nutrient density, emerge as veritable heroes in the dietary landscape of gout management. Their low to moderate purine content positions them as safe and prudent choices for individuals navigating the complexities of gout. Purines, natural substances found in certain foods, undergo metabolic processes within the body, giving rise to uric acid. Excessive uric acid levels pave the way for the formation of urate crystals, precipitating gout attacks. Thus, by favoring a diet rich in fruits and vegetables, individuals can effectively mitigate the risk of uric acid buildup and its attendant consequences.

Moreover, beyond their purine profile, fruits and vegetables offer a treasure trove of antioxidants and vitamins, essential for maintaining optimal health and well-being. Notably, vitamin C has garnered attention for its potential to modulate uric acid levels, as evidenced by several studies. Antioxidants, abundant in colorful fruits and vegetables, play a pivotal role in combating oxidative stress and inflammation, thus conferring added protection against gout exacerbations.

The inclusion of fruits and vegetables in the gout diet also yields notable benefits in terms of dietary fiber content. Rich reservoirs of dietary fiber found in these plant-based foods contribute to improved digestion, cardiovascular health, and weight management. Given the established link between insulin resistance and elevated uric acid levels, the role of fiber in regulating insulin levels assumes paramount importance in the context of gout management. Furthermore, the satiating effect of fiber aids in weight management, crucial for mitigating the risk of gout onset or recurrence, as obesity represents a significant predisposing factor.

Additionally, certain fruits and vegetables exhibit alkalizing properties, thereby contributing to the maintenance of a healthy pH balance within the body. Although scientific literature on this topic remains limited, proponents of the alkaline diet advocate for its potential in mitigating the crystallization of uric acid, thus forestalling gout flare-ups. Foods such as spinach, kale, lemons, limes, and watermelons are often lauded for their alkalizing effects, further underscoring the importance of incorporating a diverse array of fruits and vegetables into the gout-friendly diet.

Furthermore, the high water content inherent in many fruits and vegetables confers additional benefits in terms of hydration, a cornerstone of gout management. Adequate hydration supports renal function, facilitating the excretion of uric acid and diminishing the likelihood of urate crystal formation. Thus, by integrating hydrating fruits and vegetables into their dietary regimen, individuals with gout can bolster their hydration status, thereby reducing the risk of gout flares and promoting overall kidney health.

In essence, fruits and vegetables emerge as indispensable components of a gout-friendly diet, offering a holistic approach to symptom management and recurrence prevention. Their multifaceted benefits, spanning from antioxidant properties to alkalizing effects and hydration support, underscore their pivotal role in the dietary armamentarium against gout. However, it is imperative to recognize that dietary interventions must be complemented by comprehensive lifestyle modifications, medication adherence, and personalized medical guidance from healthcare professionals. By harnessing the nutritional prowess of fruits and vegetables, individuals can embark on a transformative journey towards better gout management and enhanced overall well-being.

Strategies for Minimizing Stress and Episodes of Gout

Exploring various avenues for stress management can be pivotal in controlling gout and mitigating the occurrence of flare-ups. Integrating a range of practical strategies into your daily routine can foster relaxation and bolster overall well-being, offering a personalized approach to stress reduction. Here are several suggestions to consider incorporating into your lifestyle:

1. Embrace Mindfulness and Meditation: Dedicate a portion of each day to mindfulness and meditation practices. Engage in focused breathing exercises, center your attention on the present moment, and release worries and anxieties, cultivating a sense of calm and tranquility.

2. Prioritize Regular Exercise: Incorporate regular physical activity into your routine to harness the mood-boosting benefits of endorphins. Opt for enjoyable activities such as walking, swimming, or yoga, aiming for at least 30 minutes of exercise most days of the week to support stress management and weight control.

3. Ensure Adequate Sleep: Make quality sleep a priority by aiming for 7-9 hours of restorative sleep each night. Establish a relaxing bedtime routine, such as indulging in a warm bath, reading, or listening to soothing music, to promote relaxation and enhance sleep quality.

4. Moderate Alcohol and Caffeine Consumption: Limit your intake of alcohol and caffeinated beverages, as they can exacerbate stress levels and trigger gout episodes. Reduce consumption if you notice a correlation between these substances and heightened symptoms.

5. Establish Realistic Goals: Avoid overwhelming yourself with excessive obligations by setting

achievable daily goals and breaking tasks into manageable steps. This approach can prevent feelings of stress and promote a sense of accomplishment.

6. Cultivate Supportive Relationships: Maintain connections with friends and family to cultivate a strong support network. Sharing concerns with trusted individuals can provide emotional support and offer fresh perspectives on managing stress.

7. Pursue Enjoyable Hobbies: Dedicate time to hobbies and activities that bring you joy and relaxation, whether it involves cooking, gardening, or creative pursuits like playing an instrument or painting. Engaging in pleasurable

pastimes can serve as a welcome escape from stressors.

8. Implement Effective Time Management: Organize your daily responsibilities and prioritize tasks based on importance to optimize productivity and reduce stress. By managing your time efficiently, you can accomplish more without succumbing to pressure.

9. Minimize Exposure to Stressors: Identify and minimize sources of stress in your life by setting boundaries and establishing healthy coping mechanisms. Whether it involves certain situations, individuals, or environments, creating boundaries can contribute to stress reduction.

10. Seek Professional Support: If stress begins to significantly impact your well-being or becomes challenging to manage independently, don't hesitate to seek assistance from a mental health professional. They can offer personalized guidance and coping strategies tailored to your needs.

Remember that stress management is a unique journey for each individual, and what works for one person may not be effective for another. Experiment with different approaches and techniques to discover what brings you the most relief, and incorporate those practices into your daily routine to support stress reduction and potentially decrease the frequency of gout flare-ups. By prioritizing self-care and implementing effective stress management strategies, you can cultivate resilience and enhance your overall quality of life. v

CHAPTER 3
GOUT TREATMENTS AND DIETARY ADDITIONS

Gout medications play a pivotal role in the comprehensive management of gout, as they effectively target pain relief, inflammation reduction, and the prevention of future gout attacks. Among the diverse array of pharmaceutical interventions available, two primary categories stand out: acute gout medications and long-term preventative drugs.

For the immediate alleviation of the sudden and intense pain synonymous with gout flares, acute gout medications come to the forefront. Typically, nonsteroidal anti-inflammatory drugs (NSAIDs) like ibuprofen and naproxen serve as frontline treatments, exerting their effects by inhibiting the production of pain and inflammation-inducing molecules. Colchicine emerges as another vital player in this domain, especially when NSAIDs prove ineffective or intolerable. By impeding the activity of white blood cells within the inflamed joint, colchicine effectively diminishes pain and inflammation. Additionally, corticosteroids, whether administered orally or intravenously, represent another valuable option for quelling acute gout-related inflammation.

In contrast, long-term preventative drugs assume a crucial role in managing individuals prone to recurrent gout attacks or those with elevated uric acid levels. Operating on the principle of reducing uric acid levels in the bloodstream, these medications forestall the formation of urate crystals, thus thwarting the progression of gout. Xanthine oxidase inhibitors, such as allopurinol and febuxostat, inhibit the activity of an enzyme pivotal in uric acid production. Conversely, uricosuric drugs like probenecid enhance the excretion of uric acid through the kidneys, effectively lowering overall uric acid levels. In instances of severe, treatment-resistant gout, pegloticase, an enzyme replacement therapy, represents a last resort, converting uric acid into a more soluble form for efficient excretion.

Moreover, the integration of supplements into the treatment regimen warrants consideration, either as adjuncts to conventional medications or as complementary strategies for managing gout. While supplements like vitamin C, cherry extract, fish oil, bromelain, and turmeric hold promise in ameliorating gout symptoms and reducing inflammation, their efficacy varies from individual to individual. However, it's imperative to underscore that supplements should never serve as substitutes for prescribed medications or a balanced diet. Prior medical consultation is paramount before incorporating any supplements into one's regimen to mitigate the risk of adverse interactions or effects.

In essence, successful gout management hinges on a multifaceted approach encompassing dietary modifications, pharmacotherapy, lifestyle adjustments, and, when appropriate, supplementary interventions. By synergistically harnessing the benefits of medications, supplements, and holistic lifestyle changes, individuals can effectively navigate the challenges posed by gout, thus fostering enhanced well-being and improved quality of life.

Various Medications for Gout and Their Associated Adverse Effects

Nonsteroidal Anti-Inflammatory Drugs (NSAIDs) serve as a common recourse during gout flares, aiming to mitigate the pain and inflammation associated with the condition. By targeting specific inflammatory enzymes, such as cyclooxygenase, NSAIDs effectively suppress the inflammatory response. Among the widely utilized NSAIDs are naproxen and ibuprofen; however, their administration can occasionally precipitate gastrointestinal discomfort, including symptoms like indigestion, abdominal pain, and in severe cases, ulcers. Prolonged NSAID use also poses potential risks, such as renal impairment and an elevated susceptibility to cardiovascular complications such as myocardial infarction and stroke.

Colchicine, an age-old remedy for gout, operates by curbing inflammation and impeding the migration of certain white blood cells to the inflamed joint. While efficacious in managing acute gout episodes and preventing recurrent attacks, higher doses of colchicine may elicit undesirable gastrointestinal side effects such as nausea, vomiting, and diarrhea. Strategies to mitigate these adverse effects often involve dose adjustment or concurrent administration with food.

Corticosteroids, exemplified by prednisone and prednisolone, manifest potent anti-inflammatory properties and are available in oral or injectable formulations for the management of acute gouty flares. Despite their efficacy in alleviating pain and inflammation during gout attacks, prolonged or high-dose corticosteroid therapy may engender a spectrum of adverse effects, encompassing weight gain, hyperglycemia, hypertension, mood disturbances, and heightened susceptibility to infections.

Allopurinol and febuxostat, belonging to the class of Xanthine Oxidase Inhibitors (XOIs), exert their therapeutic effect by curtailing the production of uric acid in the body. Widely prescribed for long-term gout management and prophylaxis against recurrent attacks, XOIs entail the risk of hypersensitivity reactions, ranging from benign skin rashes to life-threatening anaphylactic shock. Infrequently, these medications may also precipitate renal or hepatic dysfunction, underscoring the importance of cautious dose titration to mitigate adverse reactions.

Uricosuric agents, typified by probenecid, facilitate the renal excretion of uric acid, thereby ameliorating hyperuricemia in individuals with compromised uric acid excretory capacity. While effective in augmenting uric acid elimination, uricosuric drugs may evoke side effects such as nephrolithiasis, gastrointestinal disturbances, and paradoxical exacerbation of gout symptoms. Adequate hydration is pivotal in minimizing the risk of nephrolithiasis associated with uricosuric therapy.

It is imperative to acknowledge that individual responses to pharmacotherapy can vary widely, with not all individuals experiencing adverse effects. Nonetheless, vigilant adherence to healthcare provider recommendations and prompt reporting of any untoward effects are imperative for ensuring patient safety and optimizing treatment outcomes. A judicious balance between the therapeutic benefits and potential risks of gout medications is indispensable in tailoring a personalized and efficacious treatment regimen for each patient.

Observing and Recording Symptoms of Gout

Successful management of gout hinges upon a meticulous approach to monitoring and tracking the symptoms associated with this condition. By vigilantly observing and documenting these symptoms, individuals can gain invaluable insights into their body's response to various triggers and circumstances, enabling them to make informed decisions regarding their gout treatment regimen. Here, we delve into a comprehensive rationale for and methodology of symptom tracking in gout management:

The Importance of Monitoring: Comprehensive symptom monitoring offers both patients and healthcare providers invaluable information regarding the frequency, severity, and precipitating factors of gout attacks. This data forms the bedrock upon which tailored treatment plans are constructed, addressing the unique needs and circumstances of each individual. Through consistent observation, patterns and trends emerge, facilitating the early detection of changes or advancements in the condition over time.

Tracking Gout Flare-Ups: Gout flare-ups manifest through sudden, intense joint pain, accompanied by swelling, redness, and warmth in the affected area. It is imperative to meticulously record each flare-up, noting the timing, location, and intensity of the pain on a standardized scale. Additionally, identifying potential triggers preceding these episodes, such as dietary choices, alcohol consumption, stressors, or alterations in medication regimens, provides valuable insights into mitigating future occurrences.

Dietary Observations: Given the significant influence of diet on gout symptoms, maintaining a detailed dietary journal becomes paramount. Recording daily food and beverage intake, along with portion sizes, facilitates the identification of purine-rich foods that may exacerbate uric acid levels, precipitating gout attacks. Conversely, noting foods with low purine content or anti-inflammatory properties can aid in crafting a gout-friendly dietary regimen.

Fluid Intake Monitoring: Adequate hydration is essential for facilitating the excretion of excess uric acid from the body, thereby reducing the risk of gout flare-ups and associated complications, such as kidney stones. Tracking daily fluid intake, encompassing water, herbal teas, and other beverages, ensures optimal hydration levels are maintained, thus mitigating gout-related risks.

Joint Health and Mobility Assessment: Gout can impede joint mobility and function, resulting in stiffness and reduced range of motion. Regularly documenting any limitations in joint mobility during and between flare-ups provides healthcare providers with valuable insight into disease progression, enabling the formulation of tailored interventions aimed at enhancing mobility and alleviating pain.

Consideration of Lifestyle Factors: Various lifestyle factors, including stress levels, sleep quality, and physical activity, can significantly impact gout symptoms. Consistently logging stress levels, sleep patterns, and exercise routines facilitates the identification of correlations with gout flare-ups or symptom relief, empowering individuals to make targeted lifestyle modifications.

Medication and Treatment Records: Maintaining detailed records of gout medication dosages and any observed side effects is essential for optimizing treatment efficacy. This information equips healthcare providers with the necessary data to make informed adjustments to treatment plans, ensuring optimal symptom management and minimizing medication-related complications.

Collaboration with Healthcare Providers: Open communication and collaboration with healthcare providers are fundamental to effective gout management. Sharing comprehensive symptom monitoring data enables healthcare professionals to conduct thorough assessments, tailor treatment strategies, and implement holistic interventions encompassing medication adjustments, dietary modifications, and lifestyle changes.

By diligently tracking gout symptoms and sharing pertinent information with healthcare providers, individuals can gain a deeper understanding of their condition and actively participate in the development of personalized treatment strategies. Through this collaborative approach, the frequency and severity of gout attacks can be reduced, ultimately enhancing overall quality of life and well-being.

Taking Charge of Your Health with a Diet Suitable for Gout

Crafting a diet tailored specifically to manage gout is not merely advantageous; it's imperative for individuals seeking to exert control over the frequency and intensity of gout attacks. By making deliberate and informed choices about what they eat, individuals can not only mitigate the symptoms of gout but also enhance their overall health and well-being. Below, we delve into a comprehensive guide on how to construct and implement a gout-friendly diet, empowering individuals to take charge of their health journey.

First and foremost, knowledge is power. Understanding the intricate interplay between nutrition and gout treatment is the foundational step towards effective dietary management. Gout, characterized by the accumulation of uric acid in the bloodstream, precipitates the formation of urate crystals in the joints, culminating in painful flare-ups. It's essential to grasp the impact of purine-rich foods on uric acid levels and gout symptoms, thus facilitating informed dietary decisions.

Central to a gout-friendly diet is the emphasis on incorporating low-purine foods. These nutritional powerhouses, comprising an array of fruits, vegetables, whole grains, nuts, seeds, and low-fat dairy products, not only boast minimal purine content but also abound in essential nutrients and antioxidants vital for overall health maintenance.

Simultaneously, moderation is key when it comes to high-purine foods. While complete avoidance may not be necessary, limiting the intake of red meat, organ meats, certain fish varieties (such as anchovies, sardines, and mussels), and select legumes (like lentils and chickpeas) can aid in better control of uric acid levels, consequently reducing the likelihood of gout flare-ups.

Opting for lean protein sources serves as a prudent strategy in navigating the dietary landscape of gout management. Substituting purine-rich animal proteins with low-mercury options such as skinless poultry, tofu, tempeh, and certain fish like salmon and trout not only mitigates the risk of gout attacks but also provides additional health benefits associated with plant-based protein sources.

The inclusion of fruits and vegetables in abundance further augments the gout-friendly diet. Beyond their low purine content, these colorful staples boast compounds that actively contribute to reducing uric acid levels and inflammation, thus serving as potent allies in the battle against gout.

Whole grains emerge as another cornerstone of the gout-friendly diet, thanks to their high fiber content and diverse array of nutrients. Varieties such as oats, quinoa, brown rice, and whole wheat not only aid in gout management but also contribute to stabilizing blood sugar levels, promoting overall metabolic health.

Moderating dairy intake, particularly opting for low-fat dairy products, is generally advisable for individuals managing gout. However, vigilance is warranted, as high-fat dairy products may exacerbate gout symptoms, underscoring the importance of making informed dietary choices.

Hydration plays a pivotal role in gout management by facilitating the elimination of excess uric acid from the body. Thus, maintaining adequate fluid intake is paramount in reducing the risk of gout attacks and preventing uric acid accumulation.

Portion control remains a critical aspect of the gout-friendly diet. Even with ostensibly beneficial foods, overindulgence, particularly in purine-rich options, can precipitate gout flare-ups. Hence, practicing mindfulness and exercising restraint in portion sizes are essential habits to cultivate.

Personalization is key in navigating the nuances of dietary management in gout. Each individual may respond differently to specific dietary components, necessitating a personalized approach to identify and address personal triggers effectively.

Seeking guidance from healthcare professionals, including medical physicians and registered dieticians specialized in gout management, is indispensable. Collaborating with these experts enables individuals to receive tailored guidance, monitor progress, and make necessary adjustments to their diet and treatment plans, thereby optimizing outcomes and enhancing quality of life.

In sum, armed with a comprehensive understanding of the principles underpinning a gout-friendly diet and supported by personalized guidance from healthcare professionals, individuals can proactively manage their condition, attenuate the frequency and severity of gout attacks, and ultimately elevate their overall quality of life.

CHAPTER 4
THE SIMPLE GOUT DIET RECIPES TO DIMINISH GOUT AND FLARE-UPS

SIMPLE BREAKFAST RECIPES FOR YOU TO TRY

Healthy baked oats

What You Need

100ml almond milk or milk of your choice

1 large egg

50g porridge oats

1 tsp cinnamon

½ - 1 tsp vanilla essence

50g bio yogurt

cinnamon for dusting

60g blueberries

Method

STEP 1

Heat the oven to 200C/180C fan/gas 6. Beat the milk, egg and oats together with 2 tbsp water, the cinnamon and vanilla essence. Divide between two 165ml ramekins, then bake in the oven for 10 mins until almost set. Top each one with half the yogurt, then dust with cinnamon and top with the berries.

Vegan mushroom & potato hash

What You Need

100g porridge oats

70ml fortified soya milk

½ tsp baking powder

2 medium potatoes (275g), no need to peel, cut into slim wedges

For the hash

2 tbsp rapeseed oil

200g mushrooms, thickly sliced

1 red onion, roughly chopped

1 tsp smoked paprika

4 vine tomatoes, halved

Method

STEP 1

Tip the oats and soya milk into a large bowl
and blitz using a hand blender to break down

the oats to a less coarse texture. Set aside for 10 mins to soak.

STEP 2

Meanwhile, boil the potatoes for 5 mins, then drain. Heat the oil in a large non-stick frying pan over a medium heat, and cook the mushrooms, onion and paprika for a few minutes until softened. Tip in the potatoes and cook for 10 mins, turning the mixture over every now and then. Stir in the halved tomatoes and leave to cook for 5 mins.

STEP 3

The oat mixture should now be stiff. Work in the baking powder using your hands, then halve the mixture. With wet hands, press out one half of the mixture on a plastic chopping board to make a thin disc, like a pancake. Carefully lift it off with a palette knife and cook in a dry non-stick frying pan for 2 mins on each side. Remove to a plate, and repeat with the other half. Put the oat thins on two plates and top with the hash to serve.

Peanut butter & banana on toast

What You Need

2 slices granary bread

1 small banana

½ tsp cinnamon

1 tbsp crunchy peanut butter

Method

STEP 1

Toast bread and slice banana. Layer banana on one slice of toast and dust with cinnamon. Spread the second slice with peanut butter, then sandwich the two together and eat straight away.

Overnight oats with apricots & yogurt

What You Need

For the oats

200g oats

50g chia seeds

1 tbsp vanilla extract

550ml almond milk, or cow's milk (if non-vegan)

For the apricots

1 tsp rapeseed oil

320g pack fresh apricots, stoned and quartered

400g pot fortified oat or plain bio yogurt

4 tsp sunflower seeds

Method

STEP 1

Mix the oats and chia in a bowl with the vanilla and almond milk. Cover and chill overnight.

STEP 2

Heat the oil in a small non-stick pan. Add the apricots in a single layer, then cover the pan and cook over a low heat for 5 mins, until softened. Stir well and cook a few minutes more if needed – they will cook a little more in the residual heat as they cool. Cover and keep chilled until needed.

STEP 3

The next day, stir the yogurt into the oats and spoon into tumblers, small jars or small bowls. Top with the cooked apricots and sunflower seeds. Will keep covered and chilled for up to four days.

Veggie breakfast bakes

What You Need

4 large field mushrooms

8 tomatoes, halved

1 garlic clove, thinly sliced

2 tsp olive oil

200g bag spinach

4 eggs

Method

STEP 1

Heat oven to 200C/180C fan/gas 6. Put the mushrooms and tomatoes into 4 ovenproof dishes. Divide garlic between the dishes, drizzle over the oil and some seasoning, then bake for 10 mins.

STEP 2

Meanwhile, put the spinach into a large colander, then pour over a kettle of boiling water to wilt it. Squeeze out any excess water, then add the spinach to the dishes. Make a little gap between the vegetables and crack an egg into each dish. Return to the oven and cook for a further 8-10 mins or until the egg is cooked to your liking.

Fruit & nut breakfast bowl

What You Need

6 tbsp porridge oats

2 oranges

just under ½ x 200ml tub 0% fat Greek-style yogurt

60g pot raisins, nuts, goji berries and seeds

Method

STEP 1

Put the oats in a non-stick pan with 400ml water and cook over the heat, stirring occasionally for about 4 mins until thickened.

STEP 2

Meanwhile, cut the peel and pith from the oranges then slice them in half, cutting down either side, as closely as you can, to where the stalk would be as this will remove quite a tough section of the membrane. Now just chop the oranges.

STEP 3

Pour the porridge into bowls, spoon on the yogurt then pile on the oranges and the fruit, nut and seed mixture.

Pistachio nut & spiced apple Bircher muesli

What You Need

For the base What You Need

50g jumbo porridge oat

50ml apple juice

large pinch cinnamon

large pinch nutmeg

1 medium apple, cored and grated

2 tbsp low-fat natural yogurt

For the topping

25g chopped pistachio

3 tbsp pomegranate seeds or mixed berries

Method

STEP 1

Mix all the base What You Need, except the yogurt, with 150ml water and leave to soak for at least 20 mins or overnight, if possible. Once the oats have softened, stir through the yogurt, then divide the mixture between 2 bowls.

Sprinkle half of the topping over each bowl and serve.

Overnight oats

What You Need

¼ tsp ground cinnamon

50g rolled porridge oats

2 tbsp natural yogurt

50g mixed berries

drizzle of honey

½ tbsp nut butter (we used almond)

Method

STEP 1

The night before serving, stir the cinnamon and 100ml water (or milk) into your oats with a pinch of salt.

STEP 2

The next day, loosen with a little more water (or milk) if needed. Top with the yogurt, berries, a drizzle of honey and the nut butter.

Scrambled eggs with basil, spinach & tomatoes

What You Need

1 tbsp olive oil, plus 1 tsp

3 tomatoes, halved

4 large eggs

4 tbsp natural bio yogurt

⅓ small pack basil, chopped

175g baby spinach, dried well (if it needs washing)

Method

STEP 1

Heat 1 tsp oil in a large non-stick frying pan, add the tomatoes and cook, cut-side down, over a medium heat. While they are cooking, beat the eggs in a jug with the yogurt, 2 tbsp water, plenty of black pepper and the basil.

STEP 2

Transfer the tomatoes to serving plates. Add the spinach to the pan and wilt, stirring a few times while you cook the eggs.

STEP 3

Heat the rest of the oil in a non-stick pan over a medium heat, pour in the egg mixture and stir every now and then until scrambled and just set. Spoon the spinach onto the plates and top with the scrambled eggs.

Mushroom baked eggs with squished tomatoes

What You Need

2 large flat mushrooms (about 85g each), stalks removed and chopped

rapeseed oil, for brushing

½ garlic clove, grated (optional)

a few thyme leaves

2 tomatoes, halved

2 large eggs

2 handfuls rocket

Method

STEP 1

Heat oven to 200C/180C fan/gas 6. Brush the mushrooms with a little oil and the garlic (if using). Place the mushrooms in two very lightly greased gratin dishes, bottom-side up, and season lightly with pepper. Top with the chopped stalks and thyme, cover with foil and bake for 20 mins.

STEP 2

Remove the foil, add the tomatoes to the dishes and break an egg carefully onto each of the mushrooms. Season and add a little more thyme, if you like. Return to the oven for 10-12 mins or until the eggs are set but the yolks are

still runny. Top with the rocket and eat straight
from the dishes.

QUICK AND SIMPLE LUNCH RECIPE CONCEPTS

Roast chicken traybake

What You Need

2 red onions (320g), sliced across into rings

1 large red pepper, deseeded and chopped into 3cm pieces

300g potatoes, peeled and cut into 3cm chunks

2 tbsp rapeseed oil

4 bone-in chicken thighs, skin and any fat removed

1 lime, zested and juiced

3 large garlic cloves, finely grated

1 tsp smoked paprika

1 tsp thyme leaves

2 tsp vegetable bouillon powder

200g long stem broccoli, stem cut into lengths if very thick

Method

STEP 1

Heat the oven to 200C/180C fan/gas 6. Put the onion, pepper, potatoes and oil in a non-stick roasting tin and toss everything together. Roast for 15 mins while you rub the chicken with the lime zest, garlic, paprika and thyme. Take the veg from the oven, stir, then snuggle the chicken thighs among the veg, covering them with some of the onions so they don't dry out as it roasts for 40 mins.

STEP 2

As you approach the end of the cooking time, mix 200ml boiling water with the bouillon powder. Take the roasting tin from the oven, add the broccoli to the tin, and pour over the hot stock followed by the lime juice, then quickly cover with the foil and put back in the oven for 10 more mins until the broccoli is just tender.

Chickpea soup with chunky gremolata

What You Need

2 tbsp cold-pressed rapeseed oil

3 onions, chopped (about 340g)

3 x 400g cans chickpeas, don't drain off the liquid

3 large cloves garlic, finely grated

1 red chilli, seeded and chopped

2 tsp ground coriander

1 tsp cumin seeds

4 tsp vegetable bouillon powder

1 aubergine, finely cubed (350g)

2 tbsp tahini

210g can chickpeas, drained

100g cherry tomatoes, cut into quarters

1 lemon, zested and half juiced

15g parsley, finely chopped

3 tbsp chopped mint leaves

smoked paprika, for dusting

Method

STEP 1

Heat 1 tbsp oil in a large pan and fry the onions
for 10 mins to soften. Tip the 3 cans of
chickpeas into the pan and stir in 2 of the
grated garlic cloves, the chilli, coriander and
cumin along with the bouillon powder,

aubergine and 1½ cans of water. Cover and simmer for 15-20 mins until the aubergine is tender, then remove from the heat, add the tahini and blitz with a hand blender until smooth.

STEP 2

Meanwhile, make the gremolata. Tip the small can of chickpeas into a bowl add the tomatoes, lemon zest and juice, parsley and mint with the remaining oil and garlic.

STEP 3

If you're following our Healthy Diet Plan, spoon half the soup into two bowls or large flasks and top with or pack up half the gremolata and a sprinkling of paprika. Cool and chill the remaining soup for another day on the plan. Reheat the soup in a pan or microwave to serve.

Corn & split pea chowder

What You Need

200g dried yellow split peas

3 celery sticks (about 160g), sliced

1 thyme sprig, plus 1 tbsp thyme leaves

2 onions (350g), halved and sliced

1 tbsp rapeseed oil

50g ginger, finely grated

2 red chillies, deseeded and sliced

3 garlic cloves, chopped

1 large green pepper, chopped into small pieces

1 potato (about 215g), unpeeled, cut into 1-2cm pieces

2 tbsp vegetable bouillon powder

320g frozen sweetcorn

150g coconut yogurt

Method

STEP 1

Tip the split peas, celery and thyme sprig into a medium pan with 1 litre of boiling water, bring back to the boil and simmer, covered, for 25 mins.

STEP 2

Meanwhile, fry the onion in the oil in a large pan for 10 mins. Stir in the ginger, chilli and garlic. Tip in the pepper and potato, and pour in ½ litre boiling water with the bouillon and remaining thyme. Tip in the split pea mixture and corn, bring to the boil, then cover and simmer for 30-35 mins until the veg is tender.

STEP 3

Remove the thyme sprig. Take out a third of the veg, then purée the rest in the pan with a hand blender (or use a potato masher). Return the veg to the pan with the yogurt, and stir well. If you're following our Healthy Diet Plan, eat two portions now, and cool then chill the rest for another day. Will keep in the fridge for three days.

Vegan jambalaya

What You Need

2 tbsp olive oil

1 large onion (180g), finely chopped

4 celery sticks, finely chopped

1 yellow pepper, chopped

2 tsp smoked paprika

½ tsp chilli flakes

½ tsp dried oregano

115g brown basmati rice

400g can chopped tomatoes

2 garlic cloves, finely grated

400g butter beans, drained and rinsed

2 tsp vegetable bouillon powder

large handful of parsley, chopped

Method

STEP 1

Heat the oil in a large pan set over a high heat
and fry the onion, celery and pepper, stirring

occasionally, for 5 mins until starting to soften and colour.

STEP 2

Stir in the spices and rice, then tip in the tomatoes and a can of water. Stir in the garlic, beans and bouillon. Bring to a simmer, then cover and cook for 25 mins until the rice is tender and has absorbed most of the liquid. Keep an eye on the pan towards the end of the cooking time to make sure it doesn't boil dry – if it starts to catch, add a little more water. Stir in the parsley and serve hot.

Caponata bake

What You Need

700g medium potatoes (about 6), thinly sliced

4 tbsp milk

85g mature cheddar, finely grated

1 tbsp rapeseed oil

2 onions (320g), finely chopped

4 tsp balsamic vinegar

2 tsp vegetable bouillon powder

2 x 400g cans chopped tomatoes

2 aubergines, cut into chunks

2 red peppers (540g), deseeded and chopped

30g pack basil, leaves picked and finely chopped

3 garlic cloves, finely grated

10 Kalamata olives, pitted and halved

2 tsp capers

⅓ x 30g pack flat-leaf parsley, chopped

320g broccoli florets

Method

STEP 1

Heat the grill to high. Boil the potato slices for 10 mins, then drain, tip into a bowl (don't worry if they break up a little) and add the milk and half the cheese. Mix together.

STEP 2

Meanwhile, heat the oil in a large frying pan and cook the onion until softened. Spoon in the balsamic vinegar and bouillon powder, then stir in the tomatoes, aubergine, peppers, basil and garlic. Cover and cook for 20 mins, stirring frequently and adding a little water if necessary, until the aubergine is tender when tested with a knife.

STEP 3

Remove from the heat and stir in the olives, capers and parsley. Tip into two shallow baking dishes. Cover with the potatoes and sprinkle with the remaining cheese.

STEP 4

If you are following our Healthy Diet Plan, grill the one you are eating now until golden. While it's grilling, steam or boil half the broccoli to serve with the bake. To reheat on the second day, heat oven to 180C/160C fan/gas 4 and bake for 30-40 mins until bubbling and golden. Cook the remaining broccoli to serve with it.

Spicy chicken & avocado wraps

What You Need

1 chicken breast (approx 180g), thinly sliced at an angle

generous squeeze juice 0.5 lime

½ tsp mild chilli powder

1 garlic clove, chopped

1 tsp olive oil

2 seeded wraps

1 avocado, halved and stoned

1 roasted red pepper from a jar, sliced

a few sprigs coriander, chopped

Method

STEP 1

Mix the chicken with the lime juice, chilli powder and garlic.

STEP 2

Heat the oil in a non-stick frying pan then fry the chicken for a couple of mins – it will cook very quickly so keep an eye on it. Meanwhile, warm the wraps following the pack instructions or, if you have a gas hob, heat them over the flame to slightly char them. Do not let them dry out or they are difficult to roll.

STEP 3

Squash half an avocado onto each wrap, add the peppers to the pan to warm them through then pile onto the wraps with the chicken, and sprinkle over the coriander. Roll up, cut in half and eat with your fingers.

Vegan carbonara

What You Need

360g wholewheat spaghetti

85g unsalted cashew nuts

2 tsp bouillon powder

2 tsp English mustard powder

1 tsp olive oil

200g baby chestnut mushrooms, halved and thinly sliced

3 garlic cloves, 2 finely grated

1 tsp smoked paprika

2 courgettes (about 320g), peeled then grated

4 tsp nutritional yeast flakes, optional

320g spinach, half cooked each evening as a side dish

Method

STEP 1

Boil the spaghetti for 10 mins or following pack instructions until al dente, reserving a little of the water. Put the cashews, bouillon and mustard in a bowl, then pour over 350ml boiling water.

STEP 2

Heat the oil in a large non-stick pan. Add the mushrooms and grated garlic, and stir-fry over a high heat until the mushrooms are cooked and starting to crisp up. Take off the heat, stir in the paprika, then tip onto a plate and set aside.

STEP 3

Add the grated courgette to the pan and cook, stirring every now and then until softened. Meanwhile, whizz the soaked cashews, whole garlic clove and nutritional yeast flakes, if using, with a hand blender until completely smooth. Tip the mixture into the pan with the courgettes and briefly stir over the heat.

STEP 4

Add the spaghetti and toss in the cashew and courgette mixture until well coated, then toss through the smoky mushrooms. If following the Healthy Diet Plan, serve half with half the spinach on the side, and chill the rest for another day. Will keep for three days. Reheat in a covered pan with a dash of water, and cook the remaining spinach to serve on the side.

Steamed trout with mint & dill dressing

What You Need

120g new potatoes, halved

170g pack asparagus spears, woody ends trimmed

1 ½ tsp vegetable bouillon powder made up to 225ml with water

80g fine green beans, trimmed

80g frozen peas

2 skinless trout fillets

2 slices lemon

For the dressing

4 tbsp bio yogurt

1 tsp cider vinegar

¼ tsp English mustard powder

1 tsp finely chopped mint

2 tsp chopped dill

Method

STEP 1

Put the new potatoes on to simmer in a pan of boiling water until tender. Cut the asparagus in half to shorten the spears and slice the ends without the tips. Tip the bouillon into a wide non-stick pan. Add the asparagus and beans, then cover and cook for 5 mins.

STEP 2

Add the peas to the pan, then top with the trout and lemon slices. Cover again and cook for 5 mins more until the fish flakes really easily, but is still juicy.

STEP 3

Meanwhile, mix the yogurt with the vinegar, mustard powder, mint and dill. Stir in 2-3 tbsp of the fish cooking juices. Put the veg and any remaining pan juices in bowls, top with the fish and herb dressing, then serve with the potatoes.

Little spicy veggie pies

What You Need

2 tbsp rapeseed oil

2 tbsp finely chopped ginger

3 tbsp curry powder

3 garlic cloves, grated

2 x 400g cans chickpeas, undrained

320g carrots, coarsely grated

160g frozen sweetcorn

1 tbsp vegetable bouillon powder

4 tbsp tomato purée

250g spinach, cooked

For the topping

750g potatoes, peeled and cut into 3cm chunks

1 tsp ground coriander

10g fresh coriander, chopped

150g coconut yogurt

Method

STEP 1

To make the topping, boil the potatoes for 15-20 mins until tender then drain, reserving the water, and mash with the ground and fresh coriander and yogurt until creamy.

STEP 2

While the potatoes are boiling, heat the oil in a large pan, add the ginger and fry briefly, tip in the curry powder and garlic, stirring quickly as you don't want it to burn, then tip in a can of chickpeas with the water from the can. Stir well, then mash in the pan to smash them up a bit, then tip in the second can of chickpeas, again with the water from the can, along with the carrots, corn, bouillon and tomato purée. Simmer for 5-10 mins, adding some of the potato water, if needed, to loosen.

STEP 3

Heat the oven to 200C/180C fan/gas 6. Spoon the filling into four individual pie dishes (each about 10cm wide, 8cm deep) and top with the mash, smoothing it to seal round the edges of the dishes. If you're following our Healthy Diet Plan, bake two for 25 mins until golden, and cook half the spinach, saving the rest of the bag for another day. Cover and chill the remaining two pies to eat another day. Will keep in the fridge for four days – if following the Healthy

Diet Plan pop the extra two pies in the freezer for the end of the week. If freezing, to reheat, bake from frozen for 40-45 mins until golden and piping hot.

Leek & broccoli soup with cheesy scones

What You Need

375g leeks, thinly sliced

400g potatoes, peeled and cut into medium chunks

2 garlic cloves, chopped

2 tsp vegetable bouillon powder

340g broccoli, roughly chopped

250ml milk

For the cheese scones

165g plain wholemeal flour

1 tsp baking powder

20g parmesan or vegetarian alternative, finely
grated

1 tsp mustard powder

100ml milk

½ tbsp olive oil

65g soft goat's cheese

4 tomatoes, sliced, to serve

Method

STEP 1

Tip the leeks, potatoes and garlic into a large pan with the bouillon. Pour over 800ml boiling water, stir well, cover and simmer for 15 mins.

STEP 2

Add the broccoli to the pan, then cover and cook for 5 mins more until just tender. Blitz with a hand blender until smooth, then pour in the milk and blitz again. Add a little stock if the soup looks too thick.

STEP 3

To make the scones, heat the oven to 220C/200C fan/gas 7 and line a baking tray with baking parchment. Put the flour and baking powder in a bowl with the all but 1 tbsp of the parmesan and all the mustard powder. Gradually add the milk and oil, stirring with a cutlery knife until the mixture comes together. Shape into a log, about 16cm long and 6cm wide, and press the remaining parmesan on top. Cut in half along the length, then halve each of those pieces again to create four wedge-like scones. Arrange the scones on the tray and bake for 10-12 mins until golden.

STEP 4

If you're following the Healthy Diet Plan, reserve two of the scones for another day. Will keep covered for up to three days. Halve the remaining two and top with half the goat's cheese and half the tomato. Ladle half the soup into two bowls and serve with the scones. The remaining soup will keep chilled for up to three days.

QUICK AND SIMPLE DINNER RECIPES

Pot-roast beef with French onion gravy

What You Need

1kg silverside or topside of beef with no added fat

2 tbsp olive oil

8 young carrots, tops trimmed (but leave a little, if you like)

1 celery stick, finely chopped

200ml white wine

600ml rich beef stock

2 bay leaves

500g onion

a few thyme sprigs

1 tsp butter

1 tsp light brown or light muscovado sugar

2 tsp plain flour

Method

STEP 1

Heat oven to 160C/140C fan/gas 3. Rub the meat with 1 tsp of the oil and plenty of seasoning. Heat a large flameproof casserole dish and brown the meat all over for about 10 mins. Meanwhile, add 2 tsp oil to a frying pan and fry the carrots and celery for 10 mins until turning golden.

STEP 2

Lift the beef onto a plate, splash the wine into the hot casserole and boil for 2 mins. Pour in the stock, return the beef, then tuck in the carrots, celery and bay leaves, trying not to submerge the carrots too much. Cover and cook in the oven for 2 hrs. (I like to turn the beef halfway through cooking.)

STEP 3

Meanwhile, thinly slice the onions. Heat 1 tbsp oil in a pan and stir in the onions, thyme and some seasoning. Cover and cook gently for 20 mins until the onions are softened but not coloured. Remove the lid, turn up the heat, add the butter and sugar, then let the onions caramelise to a dark golden brown, stirring often. Remove the thyme sprigs, then set aside.

STEP 4

When the beef is ready, it will be tender and easy to pull apart at the edges. Remove it from the casserole and snip off the strings. Reheat the onion pan, stir in the flour and cook for 1 min. Whisk the floury onions into the beefy juices in the casserole, to make a thick onion gravy. Taste for seasoning. Add the beef and carrots back to the casserole, or slice the beef and bring to the table on a platter, with the carrots to the side and the gravy spooned over.

Quinoa salad with avocado mayo

What You Need

70g quinoa

75g avocado, halved and stoned

1 small garlic clove, finely grated

½ tsp mustard powder

1 lemon, juiced and half zested

198g can sweetcorn, drained

160g cherry tomatoes, halved

2 x 5cm chunks cucumber, diced

2 spring onions, finely sliced

2 tbsp chopped mint

2 tbsp pumpkin seeds

100g cooked chicken (optional)

Method

STEP 1

Put the quinoa in a pan of boiling water and simmer for about 18 mins until the grains burst. Tip into a sieve and rinse under cold water.

STEP 2

Meanwhile, scoop the avocado into a bowl and add the garlic, mustard and 2 tbsp lemon juice, then blitz with a hand blender or in a food processor until smooth. Add 1-2 tbsp cold water if it's too thick.

STEP 3

Stir the lemon zest into the quinoa, along with the corn, salad vegetables, mint and pumpkin seeds, then flavour with a little more lemon juice. Tip onto plates or into containers. Top with the chicken, if using, and spoon over the avocado mayo.

Lentil ragu with courgetti

What You Need

2 tbsp rapeseed oil, plus 1 tsp

3 celery sticks, chopped

2 carrots, chopped

4 garlic cloves, chopped

2 onions, finely chopped

140g button mushrooms from a 280g pack, quartered

500g pack dried red lentils

500g pack passata

1l reduced-salt vegetable bouillon (we used Marigold)

1 tsp dried oregano

2 tbsp balsamic vinegar

1-2 large courgettes, cut into noodles with a spiraliser, julienne peeler or knife

Method

STEP 1

Heat the 2 tbsp oil in a large sauté pan. Add the celery, carrots, garlic and onions, and fry for 4-5 mins over a high heat to soften and start to colour. Add the mushrooms and fry for 2 mins more.

STEP 2

Stir in the lentils, passata, bouillon, oregano and balsamic vinegar. Cover the pan and leave to simmer for 30 mins until the lentils are tender and pulpy. Check occasionally and stir to make sure the mixture isn't sticking to the bottom of the pan; if it does, add a drop of water.

STEP 3

To serve, heat the remaining oil in a separate frying pan, add the courgette and stir-fry briefly to soften and warm through. Serve half the ragu with the courgetti and chill the rest to eat on another day. Can be frozen for up to 3 months.

Spicy veggie pies with peanut butter mash

What You Need

1 onion (185g), roughly chopped

2 large garlic cloves

25g ginger, peeled and chopped

1 tsp ground turmeric

1 tbsp each ground coriander and cumin

1-2 tsp rapeseed oil

400g can plum tomatoes

2 celery sticks (150g), thinly sliced

1 large aubergine (320g), diced

320g sweet potato, cut into chunks

2 tbsp tomato purée

2 tsp vegetable bouillon powder

1 bay leaf

1 red chilli, deseeded and sliced

2 x 400g cans black-eyed beans, undrained

For the mash

900g potatoes, cut into chunks

75g chunky peanut butter

1 tbsp lime juice

1 tbsp unsweetened fortified almond or oat milk

20g coriander, finely chopped

Method

STEP 1

Put the onion, garlic, ginger and spices in a bowl and blitz with a hand blender to a smooth paste. Heat the oil in a large non-stick frying pan, add the spice paste, cover and cook over a low heat for 5 mins, stirring. Tip in the tomatoes, plus a can of water, then add the celery, aubergine, sweet potato, tomato purée, bouillon powder, bay leaf, chilli and beans, along with the water in the can. Cover and simmer for 30 mins, stirring every now and then. If it looks dry, add a drop more water.

STEP 2

Meanwhile, heat the oven to 220C/200C fan/gas 7. Boil the potatoes for about 15 mins, then drain well and mash with the peanut butter, lime juice, almond milk and coriander. Spoon the filling into two pie dishes (ours were 24cm x 17cm), then dot the mash over the top and spread to cover. Bake one pie for 15 mins to serve straightaway. If you're following the Healthy Diet plan chill the remaining pie to eat another day. Will keep chilled for up to three days. To reheat, bake at 190C/170C fan/gas 5 for 30-40 mins or until piping hot.

Red lentil soup

What You Need

1 white onion, finely sliced

2 tsp olive oil

3 garlic cloves, sliced

2 carrots, scrubbed and diced

85g red lentils

1 vegetable stock cube, crumbled

generous sprigs parsley, chopped (about 2 tbsp) plus a few extra leaves

Method

STEP 1

Put the kettle on to boil while you finely slice the onion. Heat the oil in a medium pan, add the onion and fry for 2 mins while you slice the garlic and dice the carrots. Add them to the pan, and cook briefly over the heat.

STEP 2

Pour in 1 litre of the boiling water from the kettle, stir in the lentils and stock cube, then cover the pan and cook over a medium heat for 15 mins until the lentils are tender. Take off the heat and stir in the parsley. Ladle into bowls, and scatter with extra parsley leaves, if you like.

Red cabbage with apples

What You Need

1 red cabbage, finely shredded

2 bay leaves

5 star anise

½ tsp ground cinnamon

200ml vegetable stock or water

50g golden caster sugar

75ml cider vinegar

2 apples, cored and cut into wedges

Method

STEP 1

Place all the ingredients except for the apples in a large saucepan and season. Place over a medium heat, bring to the boil, then turn down the heat and simmer for 30 mins. Add the apples, then continue cooking for 15 mins until tender.

Spinach & blue cheese pizza

What You Need

1 tsp rapeseed oil

2 large flat mushrooms, halved and sliced

2 garlic cloves, chopped

160g spinach, thoroughly dried after washing

1 red onion, halved and thinly sliced

40g vegetarian blue cheese, crumbled

4 walnut halves, broken

For the base

125g wholewheat spelt flour

½ tsp baking powder

3 tbsp bio yogurt mixed with 3 tbsp water

Method

STEP 1

Heat oven to 200C/180C fan/gas 6 and place a

baking sheet inside to get hot. Heat the oil in a

large non-stick frying pan and cook the mushrooms and garlic, stirring frequently, until softened. Add the spinach, a handful at a time, and cook until just wilted but not soggy. Add the onion and stir it through, then turn off the heat.

STEP 2

For the base, tip the flour and baking powder into a bowl, and stir in the yogurt mixture with the blade of a cutlery knife to make a ball of soft dough. Dust a sheet of baking parchment with flour, put the dough on top and press with floured hands to make a flat 20cm round. Top with the spinach mixture, scatter over the cheese and walnuts, then bake on the hot baking sheet for 12 mins or until the dough is cooked through and golden.

Healthy chicken stir-fry

What You Need

65g brown basmati rice

2 tsp rapeseed oil

15g ginger, peeled and cut into thin matchsticks

2 small red onions (160g), cut into wedges

160g broccoli, broken into florets, stem finely chopped

2 carrots (160g), halved lengthways, then cut into diagonal slices

1 red chilli, finely chopped (optional)

200g chicken breast, cut into thin strips

½ tsp ground cumin

1 tbsp crunchy peanut butter

1 tbsp wheat-free tamari

1 tbsp brown rice vinegar

Method

STEP 1

Cook the rice following pack instructions, then drain. Heat the oil in a non-stick wok over a high heat and fry the ginger and red onions for 2 mins. Add the broccoli stem, carrots and chilli, if using, and cook for 1 min.

STEP 2

Tip in the chicken and cumin, stir-fry briefly, then add the broccoli florets and 3 tbsp water. Cover and leave to steam for 3-4 mins, or until the broccoli florets are just tender and the chicken is cooked through.

STEP 3

Meanwhile, mix the peanut butter with the tamari and vinegar. Stir the sauce into the veg and chicken, then serve over the cooked rice.

Pastrami & sweet potato hash

What You Need

800g sweet potatoes, peeled and cut into 1.5cm chunks

2 tbsp olive oil

1 tbsp smoked paprika

1 large red onion, halved and thinly sliced

2 garlic cloves, finely chopped

6 thyme sprigs, leaves picked

4 slices pastrami, cut into strips

4 eggs

small pack flat-leaf parsley, chopped

Method

STEP 1

Heat oven to 200C/180C fan/gas 6. Toss the sweet potatoes with 1 tbsp oil, the paprika and seasoning. Spread over a shallow roasting tin and cook in the oven for 30 mins. Meanwhile, heat the remaining oil in a large non-stick frying pan and add the onion, garlic and thyme. Cover with a lid and cook over a low heat for 15-20 mins until softened and starting to caramelise. Stir occasionally; if it starts to catch, add a splash of water. Remove the lid, add the pastrami and fry for another 5 mins until the pastrami is hot and starting to crisp.

STEP 2

Bring a large pan of water to a simmer on a medium heat. Take the sweet potatoes out of the oven, add to the onion pan and stir. Add the eggs, one at a time, to the water and simmer for 2-3 mins until the whites are cooked and the yolks are still soft. Stir the parsley through the hash, divide between 4 bowls and top with the poached eggs.

Butternut squash & spinach filo pie

What You Need

1 butternut squash (about 1kg), peeled, deseeded and cut into 2cm dice

2 red onions, cut into wedges

1 tsp chilli flakes

400g bag spinach

100g feta cheese, crumbled

4 sheets filo pastry

1 tbsp olive oil

green salad, to serve (optional)

Method

STEP 1

Heat oven to 220C/200C fan/gas 7. Put the squash, onions and chilli flakes in an ovenproof pie dish (or 4 individual dishes). Season and cook for 20 mins until the squash is tender and the onions are starting to char at the edges.

STEP 2

Meanwhile, put the spinach in a colander and pour over a kettleful of boiling water. Squeeze out any excess liquid and stir into the squash mix. Dot over the feta, crumple up the pastry and place on top, then brush with the oil. Return to the oven and cook for a further 15 mins until the pastry is golden and crisp. Serve with a green salad, if you like.

QUICK AND SIMPLE SWEET TREAT SUGGESTIONS

Low-fat cherry cheesecake

What You Need

25g butter, melted

140g amaretti biscuit, crushed

3 sheets leaf gelatine

zest and juice 1 orange

2 x 250g tubs quark

250g tub ricotta

2 tsp vanilla extract

100g icing sugar

For the topping

400g fresh cherry, stoned

5 tbsp cherry jam

1 tbsp cornflour

Method

STEP 1

Line the sides of a 20cm round loose-bottomed cake tin with baking parchment. Stir the butter into twothirds of the biscuit crumbs, and reserve the rest. Sprinkle the buttery crumbs over the base of the tin and press down. Soak the gelatine in cold water for 5-10 mins until soft.

STEP 2

Warm the orange juice in a small pan or the microwave until almost boiling. Squeeze the gelatine of excess water, then stir into the juice to dissolve.

STEP 3

Beat the quark, ricotta, vanilla and icing sugar together with an electric whisk until really smooth. Then, with the beaters still running, pour in the juice mixture and beat to combine. Pour the cheesecake mixture over the crumbs and smooth the top. Cover with cling film and chill overnight.

STEP 4

To make the topping, put the cherries in a pan with the orange zest and 100ml water. Cook, covered, for 15 mins until the cherries are softened. Put one-third of the cherries in a bowl and mash with a potato masher to give you a chunky compote. Return to the pan, add the jam, cornflour and 2 tbsp water, and mix to combine. Cook until thickened and saucy – if the sauce is too dry, add a splash more water. Cool to room temperature.

STEP 5

Just before serving, carefully remove the cheesecake from the tin and peel off the parchment. Scatter over the remaining biscuit crumbs and some cherry sauce. Serve in slices with the remaining cherry sauce alongside.

Fruit-filled clementine cake

What You Need

4 small clementines

200g unsalted butter, softened, plus extra for greasing

140g raisin

140g sultana

140g currant

100g glacé cherry, quartered

2 tbsp brandy

200g dark brown sugar

3 eggs, beaten

½ tsp ground cinnamon

1 tsp mixed spice

pinch ground cloves

140g polenta

1 tsp baking powder (we used Fiddes Payne, which is gluten-free)

icing sugar, to decorate (most are gluten-free, but check the packaging)

100g ground almond

For the topping

4 clementines

140g caster sugar

Method

STEP 1

To make the cake, place the clementines in a small pan, cover with water and bring to the boil. Reduce the heat to a simmer and cook for 1 hr or until tender. Drain and cool.

STEP 2

Heat oven to 180C/fan 160C/gas 4. Butter a 20cm springform cake tin and line the base with a disc of buttered baking parchment. Cut the cooked clementines in half and remove any pips. Place in the bowl of a food processor and pulse until finely chopped but not puréed.

STEP 3

Combine the raisins, sultanas, currants, cherries and brandy in a bowl. Add the clementine pulp and mix well. Cream the butter and sugar together until pale. Add the beaten eggs, a little at a time, mixing well between each addition. In another bowl, combine the spices, ground almonds, polenta and baking powder. Fold into the creamed mixture along with the dried fruit and clementine pulp.

STEP 4

Spoon into the prepared tin and smooth the top. Bake on the middle shelf of the oven for 30 mins. Reduce the oven temperature to

160C/fan 140C/gas 3 and continue to cook for a further 40 mins. You may need to loosely cover the top of the cake with a sheet of baking parchment for the final 20 mins to prevent it browning too quickly. Cool in the tin for 30 mins before turning out onto a cooling rack.

STEP 5

To make the topping, slice the clementines to a 5mm thickness. Tip the sugar into a saucepan with 140ml water and cook over a low heat, stirring often, until the sugar has dissolved. Put the clementine slices in the pan and stir through. To keep the clementines submerged in the syrup, cut out a circle of greaseproof paper to fit into the pan and place over the fruit. Cook over a low heat for 1 hr until glossy and translucent. Remove and spread out over greaseproof paper to cool.

STEP 6

To serve, dust the whole cake with icing sugar, then arrange the clementine slices, overlapping, over the top of the cake.

Decadent chocolate truffle torte

What You Need

250g dark chocolate

2 tbsp golden syrup

568ml carton double cream

4 tsp instant coffee granules

1 tsp ground cinnamon

cocoa powder, for dusting

Method

STEP 1

Get your equipment ready (see tips below). Break the chocolate in small pieces into a large heatproof bowl. Spoon in the syrup and pour in about a quarter of the cream. Stand the bowl over (not in) a pan of hot water over the lowest possible heat and leave until the chocolate has melted, about 15-20 minutes. Remove the bowl from the pan and stir to combine. Leave until barely warm – dip your little finger in to check.

STEP 2

Get your cake tin ready. Do this while you are waiting for the chocolate to melt and cool so you're not hanging around. Cut open the plastic folder along the bottom, then cut out a disc to fit in the bottom of the tin and 3 strips to line the sides. (See step 2).

STEP 3

Pour the rest of the cream into a very large bowl and tip in the coffee and cinnamon. Whip with a balloon whisk until the cream looks like step 3. When you shake the bowl the cream should wobble like a thick milkshake, and when you dribble some cream from the whisk, the trail it leaves in the cream below should disappear in 1-2 seconds.

STEP 4

Fold the two together. Pour the cooled chocolate into the bowl containing the cream.

With the largest metal spoon you've got, fold the cream and chocolate together in a figure-of-eight motion. Don't be nervous – keep going until they are evenly and smoothly mixed and the mixture has a soft, pillowy, downy texture – you will see and feel it thicken as you fold.

STEP 5

Set the torte. Pour the chocolatey cream into the tin and level the surface with the back of the spoon. Put the tin in the fridge and leave to firm up. This can happen in under an hour, but you may need to leave it longer, depending on the coldness of your fridge (you can leave it overnight if this is more convenient).

STEP 6

Unmould and serve. Unclip and remove the side of the tin, then remove the pieces of plastic around the sides. Invert a serving plate over the torte and turn the torte upside down on to it. Lift off the tin base and peel away the plastic. Dust all over with cocoa (including the plate if you wish to be fashionable) and serve in thin slices.

Instant berry banana slush

What You Need

2 ripe bananas

200g frozen berry mix (blackberries, raspberries and currants)

Method

STEP 1

Slice the bananas into a bowl and add the frozen berry mix. Blitz with a stick blender to make a slushy ice and serve straight away in two glasses with spoons.

Coconut, caramel & pecan dairy-free ice cream

What You Need

2 x 400ml cans full-fat coconut milk

3 egg yolks

4 tbsp coconut sugar, or caster sugar

dash vanilla extract

50g pecans, toasted and roughly chopped

Method

STEP 1

Whisk the coconut milk until smooth. Measure 600ml into a saucepan and heat until just steaming. Meanwhile whisk the egg yolks with 3 tbsp sugar and the vanilla. Slowly pour the hot milk onto the yolks, whisking constantly. Wipe the pan clean, pour in the coconut and egg mixture, then cook over a medium heat, stirring for 5-6 mins until you have a thin custard. Strain and leave to cool completely, then churn in an ice cream maker.

STEP 2

To make the caramel, put the remaining coconut milk and sugar in a saucepan with a pinch of salt. Boil for 3 mins until it has the consistency of double cream. Cool, then swirl the caramel and pecans through the ice cream mix, cover the surface with cling film and freeze.

Treacle apple pudding

What You Need

2-3 Bramley apples, peeled, cored and chopped (about 250g flesh)

100g light soft brown sugar

50g golden syrup, plus 2 tbsp

butter, for greasing

1 tangy eating apple, such as Braeburn

squeeze of lemon juice

175g self-raising flour

1 tsp bicarbonate of soda

2 tsp ground cinnamon

1 tsp ground ginger

1 large egg

Method

STEP 1

Heat oven to 180C/160C fan/gas 4. Put the chopped Bramleys in a saucepan, add 100ml water and bring to the boil. Cover and cook for 5 mins until the apples are very soft. Beat to a purée with a wooden spoon. Add the sugar and 50g of the syrup, bring to a simmer, then set aside and cool.

STEP 2

While you wait, grease the inside of a 1.3-litre pudding basin. Spoon 2 tbsp syrup into the bottom. Peel and core the eating apple, slice half and chop the rest. Toss in the lemon juice and nestle the sliced apple into the syrup in the bottom of the basin.

STEP 3

Sift the flour, bicarb and spices into a bowl and add a pinch of salt. Beat the egg into the saucy apple, then tip this and the remaining chopped apple into the bowl and stir until smooth. It will start to rise a little as you mix. Quickly turn the batter into the basin, level the top, then bake for 40-45 mins or until well risen and a skewer inserted comes out clean. Cover with foil towards the end of cooking if the sponge browns too quickly. Leave to rest for a few mins, then turn out onto a plate.

Easter egg cheesecake

What You Need

vegetable oil, for the tin

200g digestive biscuits

80g unsalted butter, melted

250g chocolate mini eggs or leftover Easter eggs

400g full-fat soft cheese

150g icing sugar

1 tsp vanilla bean paste

400g double cream

Method

STEP 1

Oil a 20cm deep springform cake tin and line with baking parchment. Tip the digestive biscuits into a food bag or the bowl of a food processor and crush or blitz to a fine crumb. Mix with the melted butter, then press into the base of the prepared cake tin and chill for 30 mins.

STEP 2

Roughly chop half the chocolate mini eggs. Beat the soft cheese with the icing sugar and vanilla until just combined using an electric whisk. Clean the beaters, then beat the double cream to stiff peaks in a separate bowl. Gently fold the whipped cream into the soft cheese mixture along with the chopped chocolate mini eggs. Spoon the cheesecake mixture over the biscuit base, then smooth the surface with a palette knife or spatula. Chill overnight.

STEP 3

The next day, carefully release the cheesecake from the tin (you may need to run a cutlery knife around the edge to loosen it) and top with the remaining whole chocolate mini eggs to decorate.

Best ever chocolate raspberry brownies

What You Need

200g dark chocolate, broken into chunks

100g milk chocolate, broken into chunks

250g pack salted butter

400g soft light brown sugar

4 large eggs

140g plain flour

50g cocoa powder

200g raspberries

Method

STEP 1

Heat oven to 180C/160C fan/gas 4. Line a 20 x 30cm baking tray tin with baking parchment. Put the chocolate, butter and sugar in a pan and gently melt, stirring occasionally with a wooden spoon. Remove from the heat.

STEP 2

Stir the eggs, one by one, into the melted chocolate mixture. Sieve over the flour and cocoa, and stir in. Stir in half the raspberries, scrape into the tray, then scatter over the remaining raspberries. Bake on the middle shelf for 30 mins or, if you prefer a firmer texture, for 5 mins more. Cool before slicing into squares. Store in an airtight container for up to 3 days.

Chocolate & banana cake

What You Need

100ml sunflower oil, plus extra to grease

175g caster sugar

175g self-raising flour

½ tsp bicarbonate of soda

4 tbsp cocoa powder

100g chocolate chips or chunks

175g very ripe bananas

3 medium eggs, 2 separated

50ml milk

For the topping

100g milk chocolate

100ml soured cream

handful dried banana chips, roughly chopped

Method

STEP 1

Heat oven to 160C/140C fan/gas 3. Grease and line a 2lb loaf tin with baking parchment (allow it to come 2cm above top of tin). Mix the sugar, flour, bicarb, cocoa and chocolate in a large bowl.

STEP 2

Mash the bananas in a bowl and stir in the whole egg plus 2 yolks, followed by the oil and milk. Beat the egg whites until stiff. Quickly stir the wet banana mixture into the dry What You Need, stir in a quarter of the egg whites to loosen the mixture, then gently fold in the rest. Gently scrape into the tin and bake for 1 hr 10-

15 mins, or until a skewer inserted comes out clean.

STEP 3

Cool in the tin on a wire rack. To make the icing, melt the chocolate and soured cream together in a heatproof bowl over a pan of barely simmering water. Chill in the fridge until spreadable. Remove cake from tin, roughly swirl icing over and scatter with the banana chips.

Gooseberry cheesecake

What You Need

750g gooseberries

4 tbsp elderflower cordial

1 orange, zested and juiced

125g ginger biscuits

125g digestive biscuits

125g unsalted butter

500g soft cheese

250g mascarpone

125g icing sugar

Method

STEP 1

Tip the gooseberries, 2 tbsp of the elderflower cordial and the orange juice into a saucepan. Cook over a medium heat for 10 mins until the gooseberries have softened but not broken down completely. Set aside.

STEP 2

Line the base of a deep 23cm springform cake tin with baking parchment. Blitz all the biscuits in a food processor to fine crumbs, then tip into a bowl. Melt the butter over a low heat and stir into the biscuit crumbs to combine. Tip into the tin and press down into an even base. Chill for at least 30 mins or up to 1 hr.

STEP 3

Put the soft cheese, mascarpone, remaining cordial and the orange zest in a bowl, and mix well to combine. Sift in the icing sugar and mix everything together. Fold in three-quarters of the cooked gooseberries along with 1 tbsp of their cooking liquid, then pour this over the biscuit base. Chill for at least 4 hrs or overnight.

STEP 4

Just before serving, remove the cheesecake from the tin and put on a cake plate or stand. Spoon the remaining gooseberries over the middle of the cheesecake, along with a drizzle of the cooking liquid.

QUICK AND SIMPLE SNACK RECIPE SUGGESTIONS

Miso soup

What You Need

5g dried wakame seaweed

1l dashi (shop bought or see tip)

200g fresh silken tofu, or firm if you prefer, cut into 1cm cubes

2 tbsp white miso paste

3 tbsp red miso paste

spring onion, finely chopped, to serve

Method

STEP 1

Put the wakame in a small bowl and cover with cold water, then leave it for 5 mins until the leaves have fully expanded.

STEP 2

Make the dashi (see tip below) or heat until it reaches a rolling boil. Add the tofu and cook for 1 min before adding the seaweed.

STEP 3

Reduce the heat. Put both types of miso in a ladle or strainer and dip it into the pot. Slowly loosen up the miso with a spoon inside the ladle or strainer; the paste will slowly melt into the dashi. Once all the miso is dissolved into the soup, turn off the heat immediately. Sprinkle with chopped spring onions to add colour and fragrance.

Crispy tofu

What You Need

400g block firm tofu

3 tbsp cornflour

½ tsp garlic granules

½ tsp smoked paprika

½ tsp fine sea salt

½ tsp ground black pepper

2 tbsp vegetable oil

Method

STEP 1

Drain the tofu, wrap in 4-5 sheets of kitchen paper, put on a plate and put something heavy over the top, like a wooden chopping board, or a tray with a few tins on it. Leave for 20 mins to drain the excess moisture from the tofu.

STEP 2

Mix the cornflour, garlic, paprika, salt and pepper in a small bowl. Unravel the tofu from the paper, cut in half through the centre, then cut into triangles, cubes or strips.

STEP 3

Toss the tofu pieces in the spiced cornflour to coat all over. Heat the oil in a large non-stick frying pan over a medium-high heat. Fry the tofu for 2-4 mins on each side until golden, crunchy and browned at the edges. Smaller cubes will take 2 mins each side, larger triangles will take 4 mins. Cook in batches if you need to, adding a little more oil if the pan gets dry.

STEP 4

Drain the cooked tofu on kitchen paper and season with a pinch more salt before serving.

Chiu Chow smacked cucumber

What You Need

400g block firm tofu

3 tbsp cornflour

½ tsp garlic granules

½ tsp smoked paprika

½ tsp fine sea salt

½ tsp ground black pepper

2 tbsp vegetable oil

Method

STEP 1

Drain the tofu, wrap in 4-5 sheets of kitchen paper, put on a plate and put something heavy over the top, like a wooden chopping board, or a tray with a few tins on it. Leave for 20 mins to drain the excess moisture from the tofu.

STEP 2

Mix the cornflour, garlic, paprika, salt and pepper in a small bowl. Unravel the tofu from the paper, cut in half through the centre, then cut into triangles, cubes or strips.

STEP 3

Toss the tofu pieces in the spiced cornflour to coat all over. Heat the oil in a large non-stick frying pan over a medium-high heat. Fry the tofu for 2-4 mins on each side until golden, crunchy and browned at the edges. Smaller cubes will take 2 mins each side, larger triangles will take 4 mins. Cook in batches if you need to, adding a little more oil if the pan gets dry.

STEP 4

Drain the cooked tofu on kitchen paper and season with a pinch more salt before serving.

Triangular bread thins

What You Need

190g plain wholemeal spelt flour, plus extra for dusting

½ tsp bicarbonate of soda

1 tsp baking powder

75ml live bio yogurt made up to 150ml with cold water

Method

STEP 1

Heat oven to 200C/180C fan/gas 6 and line a baking sheet with baking parchment. Mix the flour, bicarbonate of soda and baking powder in a bowl, then stir in the diluted yogurt with the blade of a knife until you have a soft, sticky dough, adding a little water if the mix is dry.

STEP 2

Tip the dough onto a lightly floured surface and shape and flatten with your hands to make a 20cm round. Take care not to over-handle as it can make the bread tough. Lift onto the baking sheet and cut into six triangles, slightly easing them apart with the knife. Bake for about 10-12 mins – they don't have to be golden, but should feel firm. Leave to cool on a wire rack.

STEP 3

Use to make our wild salmon & avocado triangles and goat's cheese, tomato & olive triangles. The rest can be packed into a food bag to use later in the week, or frozen until needed

Philly cheesesteak

What You Need

300g steaks

2tbsp sunflower oil

1 onion, sliced

1 red pepper, sliced

1 green pepper, sliced

2tbsp white wine vinegar

8 cheese slices

50g grated mozzarella

4 soft white sub rolls

American mustard and ketchup, to serve

Method

STEP 1

Trim away and discard the long piece of fat running down the side of the steaks. Cut each steak in half and put on a baking tray, then transfer to the freezer and freeze for 40 mins.

STEP 2

Heat the oil in a heavy-based pan or casserole dish set over a medium heat. Add the onion and peppers along with a good pinch of salt and fry for 20 mins, or until the onions are golden and sticky. Add the vinegar and cook for a further 5 mins. Season to taste.

STEP 3

Using a sharp knife, slice the steak as thinly as possible and pile the slices into four portions. Heat a skillet over a high heat until almost smoking. Put one portion of the steak slices in the pan in a pile that's roughly the length of your rolls. Fry for 3 mins over a high heat until some of the steak is cooked through, with pink bits remaining. Pile a quarter of the onion mixture on top, as well as a quarter each of the cheese slices and the mozzarella. Continue to cook undisturbed over a medium heat for 5-10 mins until the meat is brown and crisp around the edge and the cheeses have melted. Split one of the rolls open and carefully scoop the meat and cheese mixture into it. Repeat with the remaining meat, onions, cheese and rolls.

Marshmallows

What You Need

3 large egg whites

13 leaves of gelatine

700g white caster sugar

1 ½ tbsp liquid glucose

1 vanilla pod, seeds scraped

sunflower oil for the tin

For dusting

100g icing sugar

4 tbsp cornflour

Method

STEP 1

Whisk the egg whites in a large heat proof bowl using electric beaters. Whisk until soft peaks form then set aside. Put the gelatine in a deep bowl or jug and cover with 200ml cold water to soften.

STEP 2

Put the caster sugar, liquid glucose and 300ml water in a large, high-sided saucepan. Cook over a medium-high heat until the mixture reaches 130C on a sugar thermometer. Be very careful when you work with hot sugar. Take the pan off the heat then add the gelatine and the water they were soaked in to the hot sugar. Take care or wear oven gloves as the sugar can bubble up and spit. Stir until the gelatine has dissolved then carefully pour the mixture into a heatproof jug.

STEP 3

Return the beaters to egg whites and whip up further until stiff peaks form. Keep whisking while you slowly pour in the warm syrup in a steady stream. Keep beating the mixture until it is smooth and shiny, then add the vanilla seeds. Continue to use the electric beaters for around 8-10mins or until the mixture is noticeably thicker.

STEP 4

Line a 25cm x 35cm roasting tin (or any large and deep rectangular dish) with cling film and brush with sunflower oil. Mix the icing sugar and cornflour together then sieve a third of the mixture into the tray to coat the inside. Pour in the marshmallow mixture, level with a spatula and leave to set for 2 hours.

STEP 5

Spread a large sheet of baking parchment over your surface and sieve another third of the cornflour sugar mix over it. Upturn the set marshmallow onto the dusted sheet and peel away the cling film. Dust with a little more of the cornflour sugar and dust a large sharp knife with it too.

STEP 6

Cut the marshmallows into small squares approx. 3cm x 3cm sieving a little more cornflour sugar over all cut sides and knife as you go. You may not need all of it but they need to be coated on all sides otherwise they will stick. Serve straightway or keep in an airtight container for up to 2 days, separated with layers of baking parchment.

Squash & chorizo stew

What You Need

140g chorizo, thickly sliced

1 onion, chopped

680g jar passata

1 butternut squash (approx 1kg/2lb 4oz), peeled and cut into 1-2cm chunks

flat-leaf parsley, chopped

Method

STEP 1

Heat a large pan, add the chorizo, then cook over a high heat for 2 mins until it starts to release its red oil. Lift the chorizo out of the pan, then add the onion and fry for 5 mins until starting to soften.

STEP 2

Tip in the passata, squash and chorizo, bring to the boil, then cover and cook for 15-20 mins until the squash is softened, but not broken up. If you need to, add a little water during cooking. Season to taste, then serve in bowls scattered with parsley.

Classic guacamole

What You Need

1/4 red onion

2 ripe tomatoes

a few coriander sprigs

2 green jalapeños

2 ripe avocados, halved

1 lime, juiced

tortilla chips, to serve

Method

STEP 1

Finely chop the red onion, tomatoes, coriander and jalapeños separately. Mix together the onion, tomatoes, coriander and a pinch of salt. Keep the jalapeños to one side.

STEP 2

Scoop all the avocado flesh into a bowl and crush with a fork, leaving it chunky – it should not be puréed. Add the lime juice and onion mixture, combining gently.

STEP 3

Add jalapeños, to taste, and more sea salt if needed. Serve with the tortilla chips.

Creamy Swedish meatballs

What You Need

1 onion, finely chopped

450g minced pork (or lamb)

1 egg yolk

3 sprigs dill, finely chopped

1 tbsp vegetable oil

3-4 tbsp soured cream

Method

STEP 1

Mix together the onion, pork, egg yolk and half the dill in a bowl. Lightly wet your hands, then shape the mixture into 12 balls, each about the size of golf ball.

STEP 2

Heat the oil in a large frying pan. Tip in the meatballs and fry, turning often, for about 12-15 mins until golden all over. Mix together sour cream and remaining dill, then spoon over the meatballs. Serve with mashed potato or tagliatelle

Peach & almond muffins

What You Need

3 large eggs

100g golden caster sugar, plus a little extra for sprinkling

few drops of almond extract

25g butter, melted

100g self-raising flour

25g ground almonds

2small peaches

2 tsp peach conserve or apricot jam

1 tbsp flaked almonds

half-fat crème fraîche, to serve

Method

STEP 1

Preheat oven to 220C/fan 200C/gas 7. In a large bowl, use a hand whisk to mix the eggs, sugar and almond extract together for a minute until foamy. Pour in the melted butter and continue to beat until combined. Gently fold in the flour, ground almonds and a pinch of salt.

STEP 2

Halve, stone and slice the peaches. Divide muffin mixture between 6 holes of a non-stick muffin tin. Top each with a blob of conserve or jam and arrange a few slices of peach on top. Scatter over the almonds and a little extra sugar, then bake for 20-25 mins until puffed up and golden. Serve warm with a spoonful of half-fat crème fraîche, or leave to cool. Best eaten the day they're made or frozen whilst still slightly warm for up to 1 month.

CHAPTER 5
CONCLUSION

In summary, the journey through understanding and implementing a gout-specific diet underscores the pivotal role that nutrition plays in managing this complex condition. Throughout this book, we have explored the intricate relationship between dietary choices and gout, delving into the nuances of purine metabolism, uric acid production, and the inflammatory processes that underpin gout attacks.

By adopting a gout-friendly diet, individuals embark on a transformative path towards better health and improved symptom management.

Embracing a diet abundant in fruits, vegetables, whole grains, and lean proteins while minimizing purine-rich foods, processed items, and sugary beverages can significantly reduce the frequency and severity of gout flares. Moreover, the incorporation of hydration strategies, regular physical activity, and adherence to prescribed medications synergistically enhance the efficacy of dietary interventions, forming a comprehensive approach to gout management.

As we navigate the complexities of modern dietary landscapes, it becomes increasingly evident that education and empowerment are paramount. Equipping individuals with the knowledge, tools, and resources needed to make informed dietary decisions empowers them to take charge of their health and well-being. By fostering a deeper understanding of the impact of diet on gout and providing practical guidance for dietary modifications, this book serves as a valuable resource for individuals seeking to navigate the challenges of living with gout.

In closing, the journey towards optimal gout management is multifaceted, and the role of diet cannot be overstated. By embracing a gout-friendly diet and adopting healthy lifestyle practices, individuals can cultivate a sense of agency in managing their condition, ultimately leading to improved quality of life and enhanced overall well-being.

www.ingramcontent.com/pod-product-compliance
Lightning Source LLC
Chambersburg PA
CBHW061034250726
48653CB00001B/85